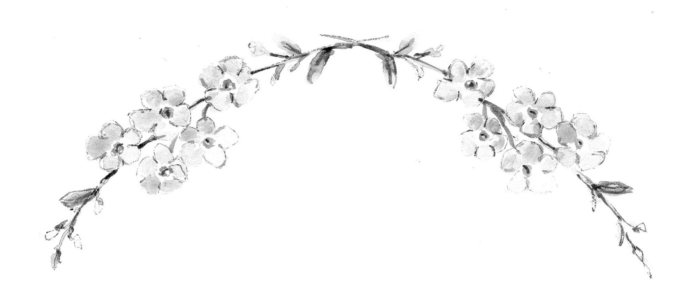

Forget-Me-Not

MEMORY BOOK

By: Dr. Iris Weinhouse, Speech-Language-Pathologist
and Nan Huidekoper, Educator

Print information available on the last page

Rev. date: 11/05/2015

To order additional copies of this book, contact:
Xlibris
1-888-795-4274
www.Xlibris.com
Orders@Xlibris.com

Contents

Dedicated to

All those suffering from dementia and their caregivers

With a special dedication to
Mary Beauregard
In loving memory

When you deal with a person who's experiencing dementia, you can see where they're struggling with knowledge. You can see what they forget completely, what they forget but they know what they once knew. You can tell how they're trying to remember.

Walter Mosley

INTRODUCTION

Dementia, of which Alzheimer's is one form, has a wide set of symptoms and is not considered a disease. These symptoms include memory, difficulty in performing tasks, language usage and even anti-social behavior. In the United States a new diagnosis of Alzheimer's occurs every 70 seconds.

People can go through several stages of dementia. This book is designed to help those with early and mid-stages of dementia who are still living at home. Some of the problems at these stages are memory issues, starting to misplace objects, forgetting familiar words and not remembering what they did yesterday. It will also present exercises to address deficits with time, being able to describe something, organizing and understanding spatial relationships to name a few. At the same time, it will give the families and caregivers a means of helping, but, mainly, it gives you the patient a means of helping yourself.

The symptoms can be in communication or in other areas and may therefore include difficulties in one or more of the following:

* finding the right word or name or understanding what is said
* focusing on a task
* understanding time orientation
* understanding spatial relationships
* being able to organize thoughts
* with non-verbal communication: misinterpretation of facial expression, tone of voice or body language

INTERACTING WITH THE DEMENTIA PERSON

WHAT THE CAREGIVER CAN DO

* always remind them how much they are loved
* give them positive non-verbal communication:
  Smile and be pleasant.
* Don't get angry with their memory loss.
* When they ask you the same question many times, don't say "I just told you that" or "I told you that this morning (or yesterday, etc).
* Try to keep their activities on a schedule (e.g meals at a set time)
* Speak in a normal tone and speak slower. They can hear but it may take longer for them to process what they hear. Along these lines speak to them in shorter sentences as they may retain less information at any one time.
* Reduce distractions when communicating with them (e.g turn off the tv in conversations). This will help to maintain focus on the task at hand.
* Encourage verbal communication. Sitting long hours in front of the television should be avoided.
* Encourage them to maintain contact with groups and people they know. Local libraries have activities that they can attend.
* They must be stimulated to continue to interact rather than sit in a chair for hours

HOW WE REMEMBER

We can use several ways to remember things – through seeing (visual), hearing (auditory) and sensation (smell, feel). It is important to try to determine which method works best for each person. To do this you can give them pictures to remember or words and see which way they remember best. Different methods can be utilized to further help memory. These include:

REPETITION:

This is best if you repeat what you want to remember out loud. For example, when you want to remember a new name you can repeat it out loud several times quietly to yourself or repeat what you want as you walk from one room to the other. If you meet a new person you can repeat their name immediately and use it immediately in the ensuing conversation.

ASSOCIATION:

Another way you can remember is to associate what you have to remember with something else. For example you are going to see a new doctor whose name is Dr. Hudson. You can remember the name is a river and this will help you recall the doctor's name as you think of the association.

CHUNKING:

This means you can remember better but putting things in groups (categorizing). If you have a list of things to remember, put them together by categories or alphabetize them to help you remember them.

HOW TO USE THIS BOOK

SECTION 1

The first section is for you to fill in your personal history from the past and present that you want to be sure to remember. It also allows you to put in photos of your family and/or friends. Use individual heads clearly photographed so you can see them better and label them clearly. Try to use a photo with an individual head for each box. Another suggestion is to paste the picture in with 2-sided tape so it can easily be removed and replaced as someone changes.

SECTION 2

This section contains 24 pages. Each month has 2 pages. On the first page you can find an exercise in an area you can work on for this month. For some of these you will need a person to work with you. You can adapt these to make them harder (for example add more words to remember) or easier (give less words). Remember you need only work on those problems which are giving you difficulty. At the end of the book you find more exercises in the Appendix.

Underneath the exercise, you will find a space titled "Things I want to Remember This Month". Here you can put in any appointments you want to make (for example medical/hair dresser/get prescriptions filled), who called you/who came visit/ where you went and so on. Putting the date in will also help.

On the second page for each month you will find a blank calendar. It is arranged so you can start the year at any time by just writing in the month and year at the top and put in the dates on the calendar as they are occurring for that month. You can enter any special days for that month – birthday-anniversaries-weddings, etc. – as well as any appointments you have for that month.

SECTION 3

This section is the appendix. Appendix A and B are additional exercises you can do.

Appendix C is a sample of a daily log that you might use to assist you to remember. This sheet can be copied and placed near you so you can write down everything that occurred that day and the time it occurred . You could write down :

> when you had your meals and what you ate
>
> when you took your pills
>
> where you went and what time:
>
> what you watched on television
>
> what activities you did –e.g. worked in garden/read/visited someone or had a visitor

This will help you remember the day. You won't feel so frustrated, if asked later about something that happened.

SECTION 1

ABOUT ME

```
┌─────────────────┐
│                 │
│                 │
│                 │
│                 │
│   Paste your    │
│   photo here    │
│                 │
│                 │
│                 │
│                 │
└─────────────────┘
```

1. Name:

2. Address: Phone:

3. Date of Birth

4. I was born in:

5. I went to school at : Elementary:

                         High school:

                         College:

6. Jobs I have worked at:

7. My spouse's name: His/her job:

8. When and where we were married:

9. My children's names are:

10. My grandchildren's names are:

11. My friends' names are:

12. Things I like to do:

13. Places I have travelled:

14. Other:

PHOTOGRAPHS OF PEOPLE IN MY LIFE

PASTE PHOT0S IN BOXES SHOWN - FILL IN THE INFORMATION BELOW EACH PHOTO

Paste
photo
here

NAME:

ADDRESS:

RELATIONSHIP:

Paste
photo
here

NAME:

ADDRESS:

RELATIONSHIP:

Paste
photo
here

NAME:

ADDRESS:

RELATIONSHIP:

Paste
photo
here

NAME:

ADDRESS:

RELATIONSHIP:

Paste
photo
here

NAME:

ADDRESS:

RELATIONSHIP:

Paste
photo
here

NAME:

ADDRESS:

RELATIONSHIP:

Paste
photo
here

NAME:

ADDRESS:

RELATIONSHIP:

Paste
photo
here

NAME:

ADDRESS:

RELATIONSHIP:

Paste
photo
here

NAME:

ADDRESS:

RELATIONSHIP:

Paste
photo
here

NAME:

ADDRESS:

RELATIONSHIP:

Paste
photo
here

NAME:

ADDRESS:

RELATIONSHIP:

Paste
photo
here

NAME:

ADDRESS:

RELATIONSHIP:

```
┌─────────────┐                    ┌─────────────┐
│             │                    │             │
│    Paste    │                    │    Paste    │
│    photo    │                    │    photo    │
│    here     │                    │    here     │
│             │                    │             │
│             │                    │             │
└─────────────┘                    └─────────────┘
```

NAME:

ADDRESS:

RELATIONSHIP:

NAME:

ADDRESS:

RELATIONSHIP:

```
┌─────────────┐                    ┌─────────────┐
│             │                    │             │
│    Paste    │                    │    Paste    │
│    photo    │                    │    photo    │
│    here     │                    │    here     │
│             │                    │             │
│             │                    │             │
└─────────────┘                    └─────────────┘
```

NAME:

ADDRESS:

RELATIONSHIP:

NAME:

ADDRESS:

RELATIONSHIP:

SECTION 2

ACTIVITIES AND CALENDAR

MONTH: YEAR:

ACTIVITY OF THE MONTH: RECALLING WORDS

You will need someone to help you with these exercises.

Try to give 10 items in a category. These can be easy ones like name fruits, colors, animals or harder ones like emotions, things that are slippery, etc. If this is too hard, reduce the number to 3-5.

Have someone say 3-6 words (whatever you can do) and you say them back to him. He/she can then ask you to say the second word or maybe the fourth. You can also say them backwards.

You can practice thinking of another word (synonym) for a given word - For example think of another word for "big" or "sad" or" noisy" etc. Another exercise you can do is take a long word and make small words using only the letters in the big word. You can purchase a book of Word Games or Easy Crossword Puzzles that are found in most supermarkets to practice recalling words.

THINGS I NEED TO REMEMBER THIS MONTH

1:

2:

3:

4:

5:

6:

7:

8:

9:

10:

11:

12:

13:

14:

15:

MONTH: **YEAR:**

Sunday	Monday	Tuesday	Wednesday	Thursday	Friday	Saturday

MONTH: **YEAR:**

ACTIVITY OF THE MONTH: ASSOCIATION

You will need someone to help you with this exercise.

Practice using ASSOCIATION to help remember words spoken to you. To practice this method, have someone make a list of 10 words and give you their association of the word which may not be the one you would choose. It might look like this: They would say "chair" –and their association would be: "cushion". You might want to say "sit" but you have to remember their word. It might be color association (sun- yellow) or parts to whole: car /wheel. To make this more difficullt use random associations (car-shorts).

The goal would be remembering 10 associations at a time.

THINGS I WANT TO REMEMBER THIS MONTH

1:

2:

3:

4:

5:

6:

7:

8:

9:

10:

11:

12:

13:

14:

15:

MONTH: **YEAR:**

Sunday	Monday	Tuesday	Wednesday	Thursday	Friday	Saturday

ACTIVITY OF THE MONTH: VISUAL MEMORY

You will need someone to help you do this exercise.

This exercise is for visual memory. Place 3-5 items on a table. To make it more difficult, increase the number of items. Study them. Close your eyes and have someone take away 1,2 or more items. Open your eyes and name the missing items

Another variation is to use playing cards. Mix up the cards and place a few on the table. Again study them and then shut your eyes while someone takes a few (1,2,3 etc.) away. You have to then put them in exactly the same place as they were in the beginning.

You can play this as a game with someone by putting half or a full deck of cards on the table face down. Take turns picking 2 cards to try to get a match. If they match remove them from the table. If not place them back face down and try to remember where they were so you can remember it when it is your turn to pick a match.

A harder variation would be to show a picture of several things happening. You study it and then, without looking at the picture tell as much as you can about the picture.

THINGS I WANT TO REMEMBER THIS MONTH

1:

2:

3:

4:

5:

6:

7:

8:

9:

10:

11:

12:

13:

14:

15:

MONTH: **YEAR:**

Sunday	Monday	Tuesday	Wednesday	Thursday	Friday	Saturday

ACTIVITY OF THE MONTH: FOLLOWING DIRECTIONS

You will need someone to help with the exercise.

Practice following oral directions given by someone. They should ask you to do 1 –then 2 -then 3 things at a time. Examples of this would be:

One direction: stick out your tongue

Two directions: stick out your tongue and, point to the table

Three directions: stick out your tongue, point to the table and clap your hands.

These must be given all together to practice remembering 3-steps at a time.

You can make this more difficult by doing the following: Place 6 items on a table and be asked by someone to: "pick up the fork; place the spoon on the plate and put them back" or "put the pen between the cup and the plate and pick up the knife".

THINGS I WANT TO REMEMBER FOR THIS MONTH

1:

2:

3:

4:

5:

6:

7:

8:

9:

10:

11:

12:

13:

14:

15:

MONTH: **YEAR:**

Sunday	Monday	Tuesday	Wednesday	Thursday	Friday	Saturday

MONTH: **YEAR:**

ACTIVITY OF THE MONTH: DESCRIBING ABILITY

You will need someone to help you with this exercise.

Have someone name 2 items (e./g shoe/slipper- or tree/bus - or magazine/newspaper)) and you have to tell them how they are the same and how they are different.

A variation of this activity is to see if you can describe an object by function or size or shape or color etc.

THINGS I WANT TO REMEMBER FOR THIS MONTH
1:
2:
3:
4:
5:
6:
7:
8:
9:
10:
11:
12:
13:
14:
15:

MONTH: **YEAR:**

Sunday	Monday	Tuesday	Wednesday	Thursday	Friday	Saturday

ACTIVITY OF THE MONTH: TIME ORIENTATION

You will need someone to help you with this exercise.

Review time telling ability on a clock. Someone needs to draw a clock face and point the hands at different times. You have to then "read" the clock and tell them what time it shows. A more difficult variation is to have someone write down different times (e.g. 3:15 or 2:00) and you have to draw the hands on the clock.

Also practice word problems in relation to time. Someone will give you a problem about time and you have to give the answer. For example: Problem: "I have to bake the pie for 1 and a half hours. It is now 3 pm. When will the pie be finished?"

"I have a doctor's appointment in 2 and a quarter hours. It is now 11 am. How long until my appointment?"

You will find other exercises in the appendix relating to time that you can practice doing.

WHAT I WANT TO REMEMBER THIS MONTH

    1:

    2:

    3:

    4:

    5:

    6:

    7:

    8:

    9:

    10:

    11:

    12:

    13:

    14:

    15:

MONTH: YEAR:

Sunday	Monday	Tuesday	Wednesday	Thursday	Friday	Saturday

MONTH: **YEAR:**

ACTIVITY OF THE MONTH: REMEMBERING

Read a story in a newspaper then tell someone what the story is about. If this is difficult have someone ask questions to help: where/when did it happen. What happened? Who was involved, etc. If you have to, refer to the story for the answers.

A variation is to have the story read to you and see if you can retain the information you have just heard. If you don't get it the first time it can be read to you again. If you can do this immediately then wait for ½ hour and see if you can still remember it. Increase the time between hearing the story and remembering it.

THINGS I WANT TO REMEMBER THIS MONTH

1:
2:
3:
4:
5:
6:
7:
8:
9:
10:
11:
12:
13:
14:
15:

MONTH: **YEAR:**

Sunday	Monday	Tuesday	Wednesday	Thursday	Friday	Saturday

MONTH: **YEAR:**

ACTIVITY OF THE MONTH: LISTENING

You need someone to help you with this activity.

Watch the news on television and then tell someone what you just saw. If you cannot remember the whole story, try recording them and play it back to hear it again. Maybe you will then be able tell someone what happened in that segment. Do the same thing with a tv show or movie. Again try to lengthen the time between the hearing and seeing the program and then describing it.

WHAT I WANT TO REMEMBER THIS MONTH
1:
2:
3:
4:
5:
6:
7:
8:
9:
10:
11:
12:
13:
14:
15:

MONTH: **YEAR:**

Sunday	Monday	Tuesday	Wednesday	Thursday	Friday	Saturday

MONTH: **YEAR:**

ACTIVITY OF THE MONTH: MEMORY TECHNIQUES

To help your memory you should practice repetition and focusing. You can do this by being aware of what you are doing and repeating out loud as you do it. For example as you put your glasses down say "I'm putting my glasses on the coffee table" several times. If you want to remember why you went upstairs repeat why you are doing this by saying, for example, "I'm going upstairs for my glasses" or when you are at the mall say "I parked my car in section 5". If you focus your actions this way and use repetition you will remember better.

THINGS I WANT TO REMEMBER THIS MONTH

1:

2:

3:

4:

5:

6:

7:

8:

9:

10:

11:

12:

13:

14:

15:

MONTH: **YEAR:**

Sunday	Monday	Tuesday	Wednesday	Thursday	Friday	Saturday

MONTH: **YEAR:**

ACTIVITY OF THE MONTH: ORGANIZATION

You will need help to do this activity.

For organization of ideas and to increase verbal output describe to someone how to do an activity like scramble eggs/fix a squeaky door/take a shower/play baseball/plant a flower. You first have to tell them all the items needed and then in a logical order how you would do the task.

THINGS I WANT TO REMEMBER THIS MONTH

1:
2:
3:
4:
5:
6:
7:
8:
9:
10:
11:
12:
13:
14:
15:

MONTH: **YEAR:**

Sunday	Monday	Tuesday	Wednesday	Thursday	Friday	Saturday

MONTH: YEAR:

ACTIVITY OF THE MONTH: WRITING

If you need to practice your writing skills do any of the activities in the previous months that require recalling words, directions, newspaper stories, etc. and write your answers instead of just saying them.

THINGS I WANT TO REMEMBER THIS MONTH
1:
2:
3:
4:
5:
6:
7:
8:
9:
10:
11:
12:
13:
14:
15:

MONTH: **YEAR:**

Sunday	Monday	Tuesday	Wednesday	Thursday	Friday	Saturday

MONTH: **YEAR:**

ACTIVITY OF THE MONTH: PUTTING IT ALL TOGETHER

Make an effort this month to incorporate all the exercises and activities you have practiced into your daily routine. Try to talk as much as possible and use the memory exercises every day.
If you haven't already been using the daily log (see appendix A) start using it now. You can copy this sheet and put it up on the wall or fridge for convenience.

THINGS I WANT TO REMEMBER THIS MONTH
    1:
    2:
    3:
    4:
    5:
    6:
    7:
    8:
    9:
    10:
    11:
    12:
    13:
    14:
    15:

MONTH: **YEAR:**

Sunday	Monday	Tuesday	Wednesday	Thursday	Friday	Saturday

APPENDIX

APPENDIX A

Here are further suggestions for activities to stimulate and help with your memory and other problems:

1. Read and explain the instructions for taking your pills. Set up your pills for the day or week. You may need the assistance of someone to help with this. On your daily log write down what time you took your pills. You can then check the log to see when you took them.
2. Make up a shopping list by putting things in categories
3. Pay a bill: read and find out what is owed; write a check for that amount; address an envelope.
4. Send an email or a card to a friend or family member. Write a note on the card.
5. Look up what's on television for that day and figure out what you want to see. If you have difficulty understanding the program guide, have someone help.
6. With someone discuss a book you've read or something on television.
7. Join an activity at your local library or recreation center. Do not sit home everyday.

APPENDIX B: Time Orientation

These exercises deal with time in a slightly different way than the ones on clock reading. Again you need someone to help you with them.

Using a calendar review the day, date, month , year every day.

Ask questions about holidays: e.g." What holiday do we celebrate in December?" Or the reverse "What do we celebrate on Jan. 1?"

Ask questions about time of year –e.g Name the seasons. What season is it now? Or ask more detailed questions: "Is it hot in the winter?" What is the weather in summer?"

Ask about "before/after" concepts with time. An example would be "Does February come after May"? Or "What day comes before Wednesday?" To make this exercise more difficult ask the questions this way: "Does Saturday come before or after Friday?"

This can be expanded to questions like: "Do you dry the dishes before or after you wash them?"

APPENDIX C

ACTIVITY DAILY LOG

TIME: **ACTIVITY**

8.00_____

9:00_____

10:00_____

11:00_____

12NOON_____

1:00_____

2:00_____

3:00_____

4:00_____

5:00_____

6:00_____

7:00_____

8:00_____

9:00_____

10:00_____

Printed in the United States
By Bookmasters